Editor's notes on biomedical publishing

JACOB ROSENBERG

Copyright © 2016 Jacob Rosenberg
All rights reserved.
1st edition.
ISBN-13: 978-1539834762
ISBN-10: 153983476X

ULTIMATE RESEARCHER'S GUIDE SERIES
VOLUME 2

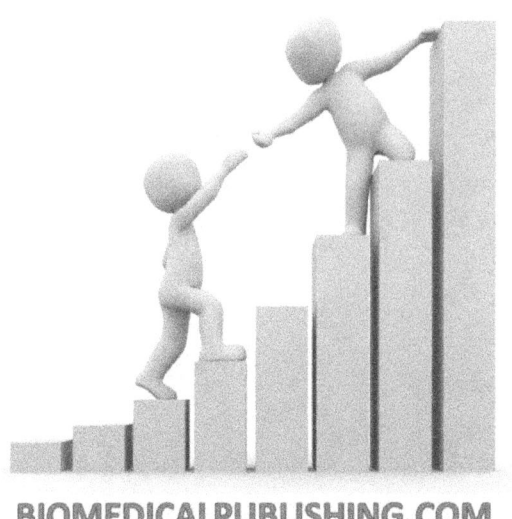

Indhold

- PREFACE 6
- INTRODUCTION 9
- PART 1: AUTHORSHIP 12
  - *The order of authors in the byline* 12
  - *How many can be authors on a scientific paper* 15
  - *How many corresponding authors* 22
  - *ORCID ID* 24
  - *Author disputes* 26
- PART 2: SUBMISSION AND HANDLING REVISIONS 32
  - *Submission of the manuscript* 32
  - *Where should I publish my paper* 37
  - *How to write a cover letter* 41
- PART 3: EDITORIAL ISSUES 48
  - *The editorial process* 48
  - *Press releases* 58
  - *How do we get all data published* 61
  - *Publication of research protocols* 64
  - *Why the paper was rejected* 69
  - *Committee on publication ethics* 74
- PART 4: PEER REVIEW 78
  - *Types of peer review* 78
  - *How to perform peer review* 82
  - *Peer review good behavior* 87
  - *Confidentiality in the review process* 91
- PART 5: CLOSING 94
- OTHER BOOKS IN THIS SERIES 96
- NOTES 97
- CONTACT 99

PREFACE

This is the second in a series of books where I will guide you through various aspects of the scientific process and how to get your papers published. In the present book I will go through different aspects of the editorial process and thereby hopefully increase your chance of getting your paper accepted for publication.

There are some key issues that you should consider when you are planning the submission, where e.g. authorship issues are very important. Unfortunately, disputes about authorship are common and may drain your energy as an enthusiastic researcher. This should be prevented as early as possible and this is why I strongly advocate for an authorship contract in writing before inclusion of the first patient in the study. In this context it is interesting for you to know that the editor and the journal actually does not care much about who becomes an author on the paper as long as the named authors fulfill the ICMJE authorship criteria and that persons that fulfill these criteria are all named authors in the byline, i.e. that gift and ghost authors are not in play. This means that you as the lead author have the full responsibility to solve potential problems before submission of the paper. That is why I have found it relevant to discuss authorship in a substantial part of the present book.

The main purpose of this book series is to help you overcome the learning process as fast as possible in order to facilitate your development into not only a top researcher but definitely also a top scientific writer. This includes knowledge about the editorial process and how your paper is handled at the editorial office. If you produce and submit a fantastic and flawless paper, then it is of course straightforward and the article will sail through the editorial process without problems from submission to publication. If, however, there are potential problems with authorship, data integrity or other important issues, then you should know how the editorial office handles this. That is why this book also covers information about problem solving from the editor's point of view.

There are numerous problems that you may encounter when doing research and writing papers and my goal is to give you tips and tricks so that you can overcome some of the most common problems that you may encounter. Of course I cannot write the papers for you, but I hope that you will get some tools in your toolbox so that you can get your papers written and published without it being a really big workload for you. For sure, there are many issues that I am not covering, so if you have a specific wish for something for a future new edition of this book or in another book, then you are more than welcome to write to me. Please use the contact form at the home page www.biomedicalpublishing.com and I will do my very best to include it in a future book release.

Introduction

Now you may ask why you should learn about the editorial process and issues in biomedical publishing. This is easy to answer because the main purpose of this book is to give you the understanding that editors and peer reviewers are real people, so you have to take human issues into account when you are in contact with the editorial office. That is for instance why it is important to write a good cover letter and also a perfect rebuttal letter when you are corresponding with the editor regarding a revision of your article.

> *"Editors and peer reviewers are real people"*

In most parts of the World it is important to publish scientific papers if you want to get your dream job. That is why issues of authorship often become relevant in the writing process and also when you are corresponding with the editorial office. In this context it may be interesting to know that most journals in fact do not care about the number of authors or who are authors on a paper as long as all the authors in the byline fulfill the ICMJE authorship criteria. This means that the responsibility of authorship disputes actually lies with you and not with the journal. Thus, you have to be educated in various issues of authorship and that is why a part of this book has been reserved for authorship issues. In this context it is good to know that if a serious issue about authorship (or other matters) comes up regarding your paper, then most journals will go to an important resource of the internet where flow-charts for handling these problems are given. This resource is made available by The Committee on Publication Ethics (www.publicationethics.org) and you can also as an author look there to be in the forefront when issues may come up.

"The responsibility to solve authorship disputes lies with you"

There is no doubt that you will be asked to be a peer reviewer somewhere in your academic lifetime. It is fun to review a paper and you will actually learn a lot in this process. Much has been said about peer review in the past and from a scientific point of view it may be true that the peer review process in itself will not increase the scientific level of the published papers. However, from the editor's point of view the peer review process is indispensable because no editor will know everything about all the different areas covered by a scientific journal. The editor therefore simply needs advice from experts and this is where you come in. You will as a peer reviewer undoubtedly have detailed knowledge about scientific areas that the editor will not have, and your advice to the editor is therefore very important.

"From the editor's point of view the peer review process is indispensable"

I have been editor for two biomedical journals for 13 years and also served on the ICMJE for 7 years. During these years it has become evident that it would be an advantage if authors would know more about the editorial process and how journals actually work. That is the main reason behind the present book and I hope you will find the information of value and help you in getting your paper accepted for publication in your favorite journal.

Part 1: Authorship

THE ORDER OF AUTHORS IN THE BYLINE

There are no set rules for the order of authors on a scientific article. However, there are certain traditions, and typically the first author will be the person who writes the first draft of the manuscript, and the last author is typically the most senior person in the group of supervisors, and all authors, regardless of position in the byline, must of course fulfill all four authorship criteria from the ICMJE.

> *"The first author will be the person who writes the first draft"*

You can even hear concepts like "sandwich-author" for those authors located between the first and the last author. This is a rather negative expression and for no good reason. An author in a middle position in the byline has fulfilled the authorship criteria just as completely as the first and the last author on the paper. They just have had different roles in the research process but they have all contributed with valuable parts to the research project – and they have <u>all</u> fulfilled the criteria for authorship.
The order of these middle-authors, or what we should call them, can be determined in different ways. Various scoring

systems have been published, which quantifies the different coauthors' contributions to the research in the belief that it should be more "fine" or better to stand closer to the first author than closer to the last author. However, this has certainly not been agreed upon internationally, and typically you will probably think that all but the first and the last place is the same and it does not matter where you stand in this middle section of the byline. In other words, you probably should not care so much if you stand on the 3rd or 4th place in a byline with eight authors. Another way to determine the order of authors could, for instance be by simple alphabetical order. My advice to you is not to focus too much on this issue. It is justified to fight for the first or the last place in the byline, but don't focus too much on the place order in the middle section. If you are very focused on a subject like this, then you probably do not write enough articles.

It is important to determine issues like this very early in the research process to avoid conflicts. It can therefore be recommended to prepare and sign a formal authorship contract early in the research process. This will determine not only the order of authors but more importantly who will be authors on the final publication. The detailed outline of the authorship contract will be covered in the upcoming book about study planning in this book series.

"Prepare and sign a formal authorship contract early in the research process"

In any case, it is typically not a problem that will involve the journal or the editor, so it must be settled by the author group before submission of the paper to the journal. As a practical advice I would strongly suggest that you make a formal authorship contract very early in the research process, and preferably before data collection begins. In this way you can avoid conflicts on this subject. If you do not want to make is this formal with a "contract" then you should at least discuss it within the research group and write it down. Send this meeting summary by email to everybody because then you have it in writing. After a few years when the paper is in the writing phase then you may have forgotten what you discussed, so write it down and send it by email.

How many can be authors on a scientific paper

The number of authors on scientific papers has increased significantly over the past decades. Years ago it was common to see scientific articles with only a single author, whereas nowadays it is extremely rare, at least in articles with original data. This is probably due to a variety of factors, but one of them is certainly that research has become more complex by often taking place across multiple disciplines, specialties, institutions and even countries. As long as all authors sign a statement of authorship, that is that they fulfill the four ICMJE authorship criteria, and no co-authors complain, then the journal usually does not care about the number of authors.

> *"The journal usually does not care about the number of authors"*

In biomedical research, we have fairly strict criteria for authorship, and these are defined by the International Committee of Medical Journal Editors (ICMJE - The Vancouver Group – www.icmje.org). There are other definitions of authorship criteria, but the criteria from ICMJE are the most commonly used around the globe. This differs markedly from other disciplines where for example in nuclear physics and adjacent areas it is normal to have many hundreds of authors on a single scientific paper. It is for certain that the authors of an article with perhaps 1,000 authors cannot all possibly have contributed with strict fulfillment of the four ICMJE authorship criteria. So the definition of authorship varies across disciplines, which is of course quite all right, but within the biomedical sciences, which is covered by the ICMJE, we usually use the classic four authorship criteria set out by the ICMJE.

The inflation in the number of authors may potentially deplete the authorship concept, and it is therefore a general attitude in the biomedical sciences to preserve some kind of rigor for who qualifies to act as authors on a scientific publication. Being an author implies that you have to be able to take public responsibility for the contents of the publication, or at least for parts of it. The newest fourth authorship criterion from the ICMJE, which was made public in 2015, is precisely about these multi-authored and typically multi-center trials.

We discussed intensely in the ICMJE in the process of developing this fourth criterion, if we could require all authors on a given publication to be responsible for all parts of the content. Initially, there was considerable disagreement within the Vancouver Group on this subject, but it landed happily on a solution that is now practically manageable. That is the current wording, which says that every author must at least be able to identify the co-author, who has been responsible for a given part of the research process. This means that all co-authors cannot be held liable for <u>all</u> the content in a given publication, but that at least they can tell who is responsible for which parts of the article. In this way, you cannot just hide behind a formulation like "I do not know anything about it."

"All co-authors cannot be held liable for all content"

There seems to be a certain tendency to not consider the number of authors of an article as a major problem. This is reflected in the fact that PubMed will index all author names regardless of the number, and that most journals and at least the journals that endorse the ICMJE recommendations have no predefined limits on the number of authors of an article. As long as all authors sign an authorship statement, and no co-authors complain, the journals usually do not care about the number of authors. In this context it does not make any sense if a journal defines a maximum number of allowed authors on a paper. In my time as editor-in-chief we once got a case report with 10 authors. This was of course a little strange, so I wrote the lead author and asked if it was really true that all 10 authors fulfilled the ICMJE authorship criteria. They had all signed a statement that they did, but I felt that it was necessary to explore this a bit further. I got the clear answer that they all were qualified as authors according to the ICMJE criteria, and then we of course took the paper through the standard editorial process. So the lesson learned here is that if the authors declare that they should be authors based on the standard criteria, then it is not the responsibility or the job for the editor to change that. The responsibility lies with the author.

All in all, it cannot be stressed enough that it is worth following the ICMJE authorship criteria and if you meet a journal that for some reason has a maximum on the number of authors, there is good reason to engage with the editor about it and get all the qualified authors on the byline. No more and no less. Once I participated in a working group where we developed international guidelines for a certain surgical procedure. We were 23 authors on the guideline publication that covered 70 printed pages in a scientific journal. The journal complained that we were too many authors since they back then (it has now been changed) had a set rule of maximum 15 authors on a paper, but I can assure you that all 23 authors fulfilled the ICMJE criteria. We had worked on the paper for more than a year with working groups, literature reviews, meetings, discussions, revisions etc. There was no doubt that all 23 should be authors. I therefore had to write to the editor and discuss the matter referring to the ICMJE recommendations and eventually the journal allowed all 23 authors to stay on as authors, which was the absolute correct thing to do. The lesson learned here is therefore not to give in if a journal has a rule about maximum number of authors. The number of authors should never be determined by a predefined rule from the editorial office but only on fulfillment of the ICMJE authorship criteria.

USE OF GROUP AUTHORSHIP

Some multi-author groups indicate a group name as authors of scientific papers. This can be done with or without individual author names, and you can see many different versions of this in multi-authored scientific papers. Thus, you can see different variations in the byline such as: author 1, author 2, author 3 and the xx-group - or author 1, author 2, author 3 on behalf of the xx-group - or simply stating the xx-group as author of the paper. These different types of indications of a group name in the byline is typically followed by a detailed explanation, that is a list of the author names in the acknowledgements section or as a footnote on the first page of the paper in print.
In the article's footnote on the front or in the acknowledgment section there are often indicated names of people who have been involved in the research process. Sometimes there is simply indicated a number of names as participating investigators, others set a "writing group" and a "protocol group" and a "data-management group" and so on. All in all, it can in such cases be very difficult to determine who should be counted as authors, and who should be counted as contributors to the work in question. This is important as an author should to be able to take public responsibility for his or her part of the content, and the determination of authors versus contributors must therefore follow absolutely rigorous criteria. It is frankly quite easy, because we have the four authorship criteria defined by the ICMJE, and if these are fulfilled by a person

then he or she <u>has</u> to an author, and if not, then this person will be a contributor. It is therefore necessary that you distinguish clearly between authors and contributors and don't mix it up by stating various group names for different parts of the work. Authors comply with the four authorship criteria and contributors do not. Authors are given in the byline and contributor in the acknowledgements section. It is not that difficult.

If you really want to use a group name then there is some help in the newest ICMJE recommendations, because they give some clarification in this field (www.icmje.org). If you use a group name, then you have to in a footnote clearly declare who are perceived as authors, and who should be seen as contributors. And do not call it something else – like committee members and so on. This is unclear. Use the terms authors and contributors. Then you can of course explain what the contributors have actually done, but use the accepted terms authors and contributors.

Now that it is simplified in this way, there is actually no need any more to use a group name as the author of a publication. You might as well list the names of <u>all</u> authors in the byline. Remember that most journals and indexing databases like PubMed do not have a maximum number of allowable authors on a scientific paper, and project contributors (not authors) can be stated in the acknowledgments section. If you need to advertise the group's name, e.g. for branding purposes, you can still refer to this by giving the name of the study group in the acknowledgments section, because this is indexed in full text by PubMed, and thereby the group's name becomes searchable in PubMed.

"There is no reason to use a group name as the author of a publication"

The use of a group name in the byline has probably gained its popularity because some authors may have thought that by using a group name then the criteria for authorship may be less than when the exact names are given in the byline instead. This is of course a serious misunderstanding and I hope that the use of group names as authors will eventually disappear. There is no reason to use a group name. Simply state the names in the byline of all the persons that fulfill the four authorship criteria stated by the ICMJE – no matter how many authors that will give.

How many corresponding authors

There has been a fairly strong demand from Chinese writers to allow for more than one corresponding author both in biomedical journals as well as registered in PubMed. This may sound strange for most people because how can you practically administer the correspondence if you have more than one corresponding author?

There are, however, good reasons for this proposal. It counts evidently much of China being corresponding author, and there is often money involved. This means that some Chinese institutions may get money for publishing an article, especially in a Western journal. For example, there has been mentioned amounts up to 100,000 US $ for an article published in the New England Journal of Medicine. So it may be very important locally to have a paper published in a well-esteemed Western journal. It is fine to have an incentive system, but then comes the interesting part: In some places it is apparently the responsibility of the corresponding author to divide the money between the different stakeholders, and it is therefore a very powerful position to be in charge of the correspondence with the journal.

It is quite obvious that the ICMJE will not be involved in these local fights, and both ICMJE as well as PubMed/Medline will only accept a single author as the corresponding author of a paper. The corresponding author is the journal's only opportunity to have a unique gateway to the author group in case you are unsure about the article's quality and it is therefore important not to dilute this accountability by allowing two corresponding authors instead of just one.

"ICMJE as well as PubMed/Medline will only accept a single author as the corresponding author of a paper"

ORCID ID

There is an exciting new thing in the World of research and that is that all authors should get a unique and lasting personal ID, a so-called ORCID identifier, often referred to as an ORCID ID. ORCID is an acronym, short for Open Researcher and Contributor ID. With an ORCID ID it is possible to distinguish between authors with similar names or initials.

In my case for instance, in a PubMed search I am called Rosenberg J, and there are a couple of other authors out there with the same name. So it is nice that instead of searching for the name it is actually possible to search for the ORCID ID instead. This is done in the advanced search option, and you then choose to search for Author Identifier in the builder. Here you then enter the ORCID ID, and if it is registered then the papers will turn up here. PubMed has allowed journals to submit the ORCID ID numbers together with the author names, and thereby the ORCID ID will be registered on the publication. This will when it is fully implemented in all journals make it a lot easier to generate publication lists, calculate citation indexes etc. Just think about the difficulty generating citation lists in web of science or Google scholar if you get married and take the surname of your spouse. If you use the unique identifier on all your papers then it will be a lot easier to follow your publication list no matter what your name changes to. Your ORCID ID will never change. Your email address may change, and even your name, but not your ORCID ID.

There are certain countries, where names are almost the same or where many people have the same surnames and initials, especially in China and Korea. Think of the more than 200,000 people in China with Wang as a surname or in Korea where Park and Kim are extremely common surnames. This can make it impossible to know who exactly authored the paper. This is also sometimes the case in other countries, so it is generally a very good idea to register yourself on the ORCID website (www.orcid.org). This will give you a unique researcher identifier, which is a 16-digit code.

"Go ahead and make that registration now"

Many journals around the World now will ask for the ORCID ID when a paper is submitted or accepted for publication, and some have already made it mandatory for the authors. So go ahead and make that registration now. There are today millions registered in ORCID. It is very easy to register, and you will have your unique identifier in only 30 seconds. It is free of charge, so do it now!

AUTHOR DISPUTES

Unfortunately, it is common that authors in the biomedical sciences will sometimes experience authorship disputes. This may of course be quite frustrating because when you have a lot of energy as a new researcher and you want to do everything the right way and you have enthusiasm and you are doing a lot of work – then it is really disappointing that you have to deal with problems like authorship disputes.

"Make a formal authorship contract"

The best way to prevent it from the beginning is to arrange everything before the first patient is included in your trial. The best way to do this is to make a formal authorship contract and then you can decide, together with all your co-workers, who will become an author in the byline on the paper at the end and who will be put in the acknowledgements section as a contributor instead. I would strongly advise that you discuss these things in a face-to-face meeting and not only on emails because you need to have mutual trust in the entire author group, and then after the meeting it is very important that you write it down and everybody agrees to it. The best way to do it is in a formal authorship contract, but you could also just send your minutes of the meeting to everybody on an email and then they should respond to you that it is OK. Actually, you can also take care of it before even making an authorship contract. By this I mean that you can refuse to work in a research group that has a reputation of authorship-problems or research ethics problems. If you are about to enter a research group, then discuss it with your friends and colleagues and listen to what they are saying. If this research group has a reputation of problems for instance if they have had research assistants or medical students making a lot of hard work and then they are not offered authorship at the end, then I would suggest actually that you do not work together with these people because it will undoubtedly create some problems for you in the end, so why not simply avoid it to begin with. On the other hand, there may be situations where you need to work together with these people because if you are entering a specialty that is very competitive and you simply need to do research in this environment, then the only thing to do is to talk about it – discuss it with your mentor and your colleagues and then write things down! This is not a signal of mistrust. It is just to guide yourself and to ensure that no problems will arise later on. So make these authorship contracts to begin with and then it will be much easier to survive this process of potential authorship disputes. In such an environment you may sometimes get the answer that everything will be solved at the end, we just make a group authorship and everybody can join that. However, as discussed above this is not the best solution. Group authorship is on its way out. It does not really work anymore because every author should fulfill the four authorship criteria from the ICMJE with no exceptions whatsoever and everyone who does not fulfill these criteria should not be included in the byline. If you use a group name for authorship then everybody in the group have to fulfill the formal authorship criteria, so why not give the individual names in the byline instead of the group name.

This was some discussion about what to do before the study actually starts. If you are in the situation where issues of authorship come up when you have finished your data collection and maybe the paper has been written already or is about to be written, then the situation is different. Maybe a colleague tries to push himself or herself in to author list, or you are told that you have to include a department head or a professor because this is the routine in this institution. This is actually a very difficult situation for a young researcher who tries to adhere strictly to common research ethics (which you of course should always do). My best advice is to follow strictly the ICMJE authorship criteria. Always. Sometimes you may feel personally that there will be names in the byline where people have not really contributed substantially to the process but that is always a matter of interpretation. You may argue that a person should or should not be included in the byline, but to be honest with you the editor of the journal doesn't really care so much because as long as all the names on the byline can sign a statement that they have contributed to the process according to the ICMJE authorship criteria, then the journal will be satisfied given that no conflicts come up.

"The editor of the journal doesn't really care as long as the ICMJE criteria are followed"

So, my advice to you will be also not to care so much if all the persons have fulfilled the authorship criteria formally. Then it does not really matter so much if one person has done more than another person. Therefore, don't worry too much as long as you can sign that all persons in the byline have fulfilled the four authorship criteria. You therefor have to make sure that this is the case. This means typically that you, as the lead researcher on the project, have to involve all these potential authors according to the authorship criteria including giving them the opportunity to give critical revision to the manuscript. So, don't think so much about it – just be sure that you have done your part and that all fulfill the criteria.

The real problem exists if a person is put in the byline and if he or she does not fulfill the criteria, or the opposite situation where a person is not put in the byline but he or she does fulfill the criteria. Then it is a matter of gift authorship or ghost authorship and in this situation you need to stand up and refuse to let it pass. So what can you actually do in this situation? The best thing to do is to talk with your senior advisor, your mentor in the research group, and try to find a solution. If this does not help you may take the problem to the head of department or the dean of the faculty or something like that, but if you do that I would advise you to tell your scientific advisor that you are going to do that before you actually do it. Sometimes that itself will facilitate the process and then you will hopefully have these ghost- or gift-authors problems solved. If you are in the unlucky situation that you are not able to solve the problem either with your scientific advisor or the head of the department or whoever you can talk to about it – then you should think carefully if you should withdraw from the paper yourself. If there is some kind of misconduct then that will adhere to you as a researcher for the rest of your life. So, think carefully about it and you may decide to withdraw yourself.

"Solve the problems before they arise"

Thus, my best advice is to try to solve the problems actually before they arise. This means make the arrangements before the first patient is included, preferably by making an authorship contract, and if you experience authorship problems that looks a little like misconduct then you have to take it quite seriously. Talk with your mentor about it, perhaps talk to the head of department or the dean, and then at the end if this does not solve the problem then perhaps you should yourself withdraw from the paper and actually find another research group.

Hopefully everything will work out and of course I would say that in absolutely most cases there are no problems at all. Keep up the good spirit and make good research!

Part 2: Submission and handling revisions

SUBMISSION OF THE MANUSCRIPT

The submission of a manuscript is not at all an exact science. You can compose your cover letter in differently ways and that is an important part of the submission process. Thus, you have to correspond with the editor and this is a thing that I would like to underline for you. The editor is actually a human being, so you have to of course be polite in the cover letter, but you can also have a dialogue with the editor about different things in your manuscript.

The most important thing when you submit your paper is to follow "The Instructions for Authors". This is self-evident, but very often the authors do not comply with the instructions for authors on the journal's website even though it should be an easy task to do that. Simply get the instructions for authors and follow them to the exact point. However, there are also some unwritten rules. You have to be polite, not too polite and not too humble, but you should write in a good tone and never ever be angry with the editor.

"Follow instructions for authors"

The submission is nowadays always done electronically through a manuscript system on the Internet. You will have to submit a cover letter, which is a personal letter from you as an author to the editor, where you will explain why they should consider your paper for this specific journal. Then you will have to make a separate title page. Very often the journals want a separate title page meaning a title page in a separate word file. The reason for this is because most journals have some kind of blinded peer-review process, so they will not want to send your paper including the title page to their peer reviewer. Then the manuscript will follow in a separate file and not including the figures, because the figures will also have to be submitted in separate files – one figure in each file. Most journals will want tables included in the manuscript Word file, but not the figures.

Most journals will have some kind of an author declaration form that you have to fill out and this is typically a form saying that you have complied with the authorship requirements from the ICMJE. Some of the bigger journals will also want your research protocol, but that is sometimes not with the initial submission but later in the editorial process. Therefore, do not submit your protocol to begin with unless it is specifically stated in the instructions for authors. Some journals will also want submission of a check-list, for instance if you have made a randomized clinical trial, then you should of course follow the CONSORT statement. This is a guideline telling you how to write your paper and you can find it on the equator-network.org website. Many journals will want this check list also in the initial submission but you have to, again, look carefully in the instructions to authors to know what you have to do.

"Silence from the editorial office is actually a good sign"

When your paper now has been submitted then it will reach the editorial office. This means it will not reach the editor yet, but it will most often reach a secretariat where they will check your paper for length and other requirements of style. If they accept your paper for the editorial process, then it will go to the editor. The editor will read your paper, not in detail, not sentence for sentence maybe, but he or she will read the paper and then decide if it should go out for peer review or if he or she will reject it immediately. Most journals get way too many papers submitted so there is a process here in the beginning of the entire editorial process, where papers are rejected without peer review. Thus, if you have submitted your paper and do not hear from the editorial office within a few weeks, then it is actually a good sign, because it very often means that your paper has passed this initial rejection mechanism and has been sent out for external peer review. This is a positive sign. Now the paper goes out for peer review and when it comes back it goes to the editor again and the editor will read the peer reviewer(s) comments and read your paper again and then send it to you. At this point the paper is either rejected or you get the chance to correct some of the things that the peer reviewer(s) has pointed out and then re-submit your paper again.

This can be done several times meaning that you can have your paper back and forth between you and the editor and the peer reviewer maybe three or four times before it is finally rejected or accepted for publication. However, the typical situation is only one round of corrections and then you get the verdict of acceptance or rejection. If you are so lucky that the paper has been accepted finally, then it most often will go to a technical editor or a copywriter that will correct your language and grammar. After this it typically goes to typesetting and then you will get a proof by email. This is a file, typically a pdf-file, where you will have to read it very carefully because this is the last chance you will get to correct typos or other errors in your paper. At this point you do not make substantial changes because if you do that, then the whole process has to start over again. Then it goes back to the editor; perhaps it goes out for a new peer review and so on. Thus, at the proof stage it is only minor typos that can be corrected and nothing else.

"Epub ahead of print"

When the paper after proof acceptance goes back to the editor or the editorial office, then it will in many journals be made available on the Internet as "epub ahead of print" meaning that the pdf file can be accessed but the article has not yet been assigned to a journal issue. The typical reference to such a paper is that it is "in press", even though it may already have a DOI (digital object identifier) address. The final reference for the article is given when it appears in a journal issue (in print and/or electronically) with a volume and an issue number. It can be discussed when the paper is formally published. Most journals regard the first electronic publication to be the formal first publication even though the article may not yet have the full reference assigned with volume and issue number as well as page numbers. Some journals do not use traditional pagination and instead the papers are assigned an article number. This is used by an increasing number of journals, e.g. the BMJ and the Danish Medical Journal. If such a system is used, then the first electronic publication will not at a later stage change the layout of the reference so in a way it is an easier system to administer and it shortens the time from acceptance to final publication.

Where should I publish my paper

When you are writing for publication an important question is where to submit your paper. Which journal should you aim for? The question often arises quite late in the writing process and this is not optimal. So my advice to you is to think about your target journal as early as possible in the research process. Actually already when you are planning your study you should have some thoughts about your target journal because this will sometimes make your design of the study a little bit different or you may include other or additional secondary outcome parameters. Therefore, think about it as early as possible.

> *"Think about your target journal as early as possible in the research process"*

If you have finished data collection in the study and have not decided on your target journal yet, then you should at least decide it before you write your paper because the writing of the paper is different in different journals. If you for instance aim for one of the big weekly general medical journals like New England Journal of Medicine or Lancet, then the article should be quite brief and more to the point compared with a specialty journal that will more often allow longer articles giving more details about the methods and a more lengthy discussion section.

When you consider a possible journal for publication of your article, then the most important question you should ask yourself is "what is the target audience for this article?" Is the target audience only specialists then of course you should not go for a general medical journal, and if the target audience is more or less all health professionals around the world then the appropriate target journal would be a big medical general journal. That is why it is very important to consider your target audience and preferably as early as possible in the research process. After this question has been answered, then you should find the relevant journal to submit to. In this process the normal thing and the advisable thing is to go into a dialogue with your scientific supervisor for the research project, because he or she is more experienced than you are and they have a better overview of the possibilities, meaning what journals you can submit to.

"Who is your target audience?"

After you have decided on maybe a few relevant journals that you can consider, then go the journals' websites, read carefully the instruction for authors and also browse through previous issues of the journal to see if your article will fit in or if you should choose another place to submit to. There is often also some considerations about journal impact factors that can be find at the Journal

Citation Reports website or at other places on the Internet. Researchers would like to publish in a journal with as high impact factor as possible, but just a word of caution here. The most important thing to consider is still the target audience. This will better determine the right journal for your article.

> *"The target audience will determine the right journal for your article"*

There is also a consideration about whether you should publish in an open access journal or in a traditional journal, because an open access journal will always charge you a fee and you should ask your supervisor before submission if there is funding available to do that. If you have the funding, my personal opinion is that an open access journal is preferable because then the audience will automatically be larger because everybody will have access to read your paper. On the other hand, if you do not have funding for an open access publication fee, then of course you should not go for such a journal. Thus, this is primarily an economical consideration. This issue is a matter of intense discussion among editors around the globe, but my personal opinion is that if at all possible I think it is a good thing to make the study publicly available to all readers and not only to those who pay.
So after all these factors have been taken into account you can probably make a list of three or four possible target

journals. You can list them on your own computer or your own notes and then you already now have your list of journals where you will submit to if for instance the first one will turn you down and the second and third and so on. Then you have already decided on the list of journals that will come into question.

This was all I had to say about where to submit your paper and as you can see it is a process where you will be in close dialogue with your scientific supervisor, and then you will decide considering all the different factors involved.

How to write a cover letter

When you have written your paper then it is time to write the cover letter to the journal. Every article must be accompanied by a letter to the editor and that is a so-called cover letter. This is a personal letter to the editor in which the authors have the opportunity to explain why you believe that the manuscript has an important message to the readers of that specific journal. It is a sales pitch but it is important not to exaggerate. Be brief and give your content and the message and why you have chosen the current journal for publication of your article. Don't write too long a cover letter because editors are busy people. Keep it short and to the point. There is no need to exaggerate and especially no need to lie of course and try to persuade the editor. The journal will see the importance of the manuscript if it is present. However, it is important to realize that it is a real person who will read the cover letter at the other end, so if you cannot explain to the editor why the article should be published, then probably the readers will not understand it either.

> *"Every article must be accompanied by a cover letter to the editor"*

You should be able in very few sentences to explain to the editor why he or she should accept your paper. The editor receives articles from a variety of disciplines and the editor can obviously not be an expert in all areas. It is therefore necessary to include a brief explanation of why this particular article is really good. It is a good idea to spend some time writing this letter. It is actually read by the editor and you have the opportunity to explain to the editor why this article should be published.

> *"You have the opportunity to explain to the editor why this article should be published"*

There are some common phrases that you typically will put in your cover letter and they are for instance: "Please find enclosed our manuscript entitled … by these and these authors, which we would like to submit for publication as an original paper in this and this journal. To our knowledge this is the first report showing this and this … We believe our findings will appeal to the readership of your journal because … Please address all correspondence to … (give your name), and we look forward to hearing from you at your earliest convenience". It is typical also to include a few more legal type sentences at the end such as for instance: "We confirm, that this manuscript has not been published elsewhere, and is not under consideration by another journal. All authors have approved the final version of the manuscript and agree with submission to this and this

Journal. All authors comply with the ICMJE authorship criteria and the conflicts of interest are given in the enclosed conflict of interest forms (if that is required by the journal)."

This is a way to compose your cover letter in a rather standard fashion, but spend some time on it because it pays off in the end.

Handling revisions

When you get a response from the journal, typically within 2-3 months from submission, then it can either be rejection, acceptance after revision, or acceptance without revision. The latter is a rare event, so most often you will get the chance to resubmit after a rewrite guided by comments from the editor as well as from one or more peer reviewers.

It is important in the revision phase that you do not ignore the demand for changes by the editor. If the editor wants something to be changed I can assure you, just a good advice, make the changes, because if you do not make these changes, then the paper will most likely be rejected. There may be other demands for revision than the ones from the editor and these are the ones from the peer reviewer(s). There can easily be up to four peer reviewers but many journals use only one or two. They will all give their comments so there may be quite a lot to correct in a revision. The mindset now that you should take is to correct as much as possible of the points of critique from the peer reviewers. The comments from the editor should all be followed, and the comments from the reviewers should result in as many changes as you can possibly make because that will ensure that your paper will finally be accepted. If there are suggestions for changes that are simply impossible to comply with, then you can also argue against them in your answers in your rebuttal letter to the editor. This can be OK, but if you for instance have 20 possible changes asked by the reviewer, then it is not OK to only correct 10 of them. That is simply not enough. You have to correct at least 80-90% of the suggested changes in order for your paper to get accepted for publication. That is at least the typical scenario.

"Do not ignore the demand for changes"

The rebuttal letter to the editor is a personal letter. You can therefore make it personal by saying "Dear professor x" or "Dear editor". You write something like "Thank you for reviewing our paper. We are very happy that we can correct it", and so on. Then you will give a point by point list for all the suggested changes by the peer reviewers and the best way to do that is to simply copy-paste the text from the peer reviewer comments directly into your letter and for each point you will write your answer including a statement of what has been changed in the manuscript. In the manuscript itself, your changes have to be highlighted, for instance with track-changes in Word or maybe in another color than black. It has to be an easy job for the editor to see the changes.

When you submit the revised manuscript, you will typically submit the revised manuscript with visible changes together with a detailed point-by-point rebuttal letter explaining all the changes. Most often you do not have to resubmit the original version of the manuscript since this will already be available in the electronic manuscript system. Hopefully your paper will now be accepted for publication and this is a great day, which has to be celebrated. However, if the paper is rejected it is not the end of the World of course. There are thousands of journals out there, so your paper will eventually be accepted somewhere if it has a reasonable level of quality.

"You will typically submit the revised manuscript with visible changes together with a detailed point-by-point rebuttal letter explaining all the changes"

Do not try to appeal a rejection because most often it will not lead to anything positive. If they say no to you it is a no. When you now want to submit your paper to another journal, remember to submit a clean manuscript to the new journal. No changes, no comments, and especially not the name of the former journal in the letterhead of the cover letter. That is really embarrassing. Take into consideration only the most obvious errors pointed out by the peer reviewers from the first journal because that will increase the quality of your paper and then submit it to another journal. You will now get other editors and other peer reviewers and they may be more positive then the first ones. So, there is no reason to cry, no reason to throw your paper away, absolutely not. Therefore, correct it with the most obvious changes that need to be made and then send it to another journal as fast as you can.

Part 3: Editorial issues

THE EDITORIAL PROCESS

This chapter will discuss the editorial process meaning what happens with your manuscript after you have submitted it to the journal or the editorial office. The first thing that you should consider is to submit the correct files to the journal. It means that in the electronic manuscript system you have to fill out all the required fields and then submit the required files to the journal. You also have to submit a cover letter. The cover letter is the letter that will follow your manuscript and where you will explain to the editor why your paper is fantastic and why they should consider it for publication. The cover letter most often is typed into the electronic manuscript system into a special field so you do not normally submit a formal cover letter as a word-file, you simply copy-paste your text from your cover letter Word file into this special field in the manuscript system. Most journals want a separate title page, because if you split the title page from the manuscript itself, then it is much easier for the journal to perform blinded peer review because then they will only send the manuscript text file without the title page to the peer reviewers. Then the manuscript file itself, typically a Word file, has to be uploaded to the system. The manuscript file will most often also have the tables, the references, and the legends to tables and figures, whereas the figures are uploaded as separate files. Most journals also require some kind of an authorship declaration form where all the authors have signed a statement that they fulfill the ICMJE authorship criteria. Some journals also at this point require some kind of copyright transfer to the journal, or actually to the publisher, but other journals they will get that later in the editorial process if the paper gets accepted for publication. Some of the big journals would also like you to submit the research protocol as well as the statistical analysis plan if you have performed a large randomized clinical trial. Not all journals want that, but it is a possibility in some journals. You can also at this point submit additional files that you intend to be published as web-only material, but again some journals will want that at a later stage. Then, some journals also like to have the checklists from for instance the PRISMA statement or the CONSORT statement. These checklists also can be submitted together with your manuscript whereas other journals do not like that. So check the author guidelines thoroughly and then you can see exactly what to submit. If in doubt you can always submit everything.

Separate files to submit (depending on the journal):
- **Title page**
- **The manuscript file (typically including tables)**
- **The figures (one in each file)**
- **Authorship declaration form**
- **Copyright transfer**
- **Research protocol**

- **Statistical analysis plan**
- **Additional files for web-only**
- **PRISMA or CONSORT checklist**

The next thing that happens is that your manuscript is checked at the editorial office and that is typically done not by the editor himself or herself but by a secretary or an editorial assistant. They will check your manuscript for errors, for missing files, or for missing sections. You cannot imagine how badly manuscripts can be submitted. Sometimes the whole reference list is missing and so on. So, this formal check is done by the editorial office in the initial assessment. This also includes the check for length because most journals have some kind of limit for the length of the manuscript. When this is OK the manuscript will be made available to the editor in the electronic system (he or she can typically not see the submission before it is released by the assistant) and then the editor, typically the editor in chief but it can also be an assistant editor, will check the manuscript if it is within the scope of the journal. This is probably the most important assessment. If the manuscript fulfills the scope of the journal then the editor can decide if your manuscript will be immediately rejected or if it can move on in the editorial process. In this initial check by the editor or the editor in chief he or she also often looks at the language, if it is extremely bad language which grammar and speling errors. If this is the case then it will be returned to the author and asked for improvement before re-submission. At this point it is also an issue if the journal has covered exactly the same topic recently and this is something that the editor or editor in chief will know of course. Then it may be the situation that the journal does not want to publish another article on the same topic so close to the former one. So that could also be a reason for initial rejection. Then the editor will of course check if there are any potential legal issues, for instance if the article will speak very badly about a specific product or something like that, then of course it has to be substantiated by very good evidence in the paper. Otherwise there may be legal consequences and that's also the responsibility of the editor to check that. Finally, of course a human trial has to be approved by an ethics committee and a trial has to be registered in a public database before inclusion of the first patient, and the editor also checks this. If it is not fulfilled, then of course without any doubt the paper will be rejected immediately.

> *"The editor will check if the manuscript is within the scope of the journal"*

So after this initial assessment by the editor then the paper should go on to peer review. If they decide to send out the paper for peer review then the question now comes up "who should be chosen for peer review"? This process is of course different from journal to journal. Most often in the manuscript system there will be some kind of a pool of peer reviewers that the editors most often use and they are divided according to their fields of expertise. If there are no reviewers available for this specific paper in the system already then the authors may have suggested some reviewers and the editor may choose to follow these suggestions or may choose specifically not to follow these suggestions. It is not a guarantee that you will get these reviewers if you have suggested certain names in your manuscript submission. If at this point there are still no reviewers available for the editor, then the editor may choose to look in the manuscript itself in the reference list for names on previously published papers that could be relevant, meaning that the editor can find experts that may be potential reviewers for this specific paper. If this is still not enough then it is possible to do a simple search on PubMed and then find potential reviewers, and finally if this also not solves the problem, then the editor may choose names from his or her own surroundings, colleagues or network.

> *"You may suggest specific reviewers but you cannot be sure that these suggestions are followed"*

Now the peer reviewers have been chosen and the paper will in the manuscript system be forwarded to one, two or three peer reviewers depending on the journal and they will be asked if they can review this paper. The email that they receive is a standard email, meaning that it is generated by the system and it is quite rare that the editor will write a specific message or personal message for the individual peer reviewer in this email. Then there is a waiting time. You cannot see this process when you log-on to the manuscript system as an author. It will just show that peer reviewers have not been selected yet, although of course they have been selected, but they have not agreed to review the paper yet. Once they agree then you can see when you log-on that the paper is out for peer review. That is why there may be a long waiting time in this phase because the peer reviewers may not answer right away or they do not want to review the paper or they may even be on vacation. That is why the waiting time at this stage is not because the editors are sleeping. It is simply because they are trying to find peer reviewers. Then, when the peer reviewers accept to review the paper, then they are given a time frame to do that, typically 2-3 weeks or something like that, again depending on the journal.

> *"The waiting time is not because the editors are sleeping"*

The reviewers respond to the editorial office in a specific form in the manuscript system where they first of all recommend if the paper should be rejected, accepted with major changes, accepted with minor changes, or accepted as it is. Then they can write some confidential comments to the editor and these comments are not available for the authors. Here typically they will write if they suspect plagiarism or if there are some political or other aspects that should be taken care of by the editor. Also they can substantiate their recommendations for rejection or acceptance in this specific field in the manuscript system. In another field they give the comments to the authors and this is what you see when you get your feedback email from the editorial office. You will see a list of comments from the peer reviewers and these are written here by the peer reviewers in the manuscript system. Now, when the editor is ready to look at your paper he or she will look at the paper again, of course read it, and look at the peer reviewers' comments, both the comments for authors and the confidential comments for the editor.

"The reviewers will give confidential comments to the editor and reviewer comments to the author"

At this point it is decided what will happen with the paper. If it is accepted with changes meaning that you get a chance as an author to correct some details in the manuscript, then an email is again generated by the electronic manuscript system and in this email the peer reviewers' comments are copied automatically in the bottom of the text. It is normal practice that the editor will read these peer reviewer comments in very much detail and also change them a little sometimes. For instance if the peer reviewer has written that you should delete figure one or something like that and if the editor does not agree with that, then it is the editor who will change that recommendation even though it is stated in the comments from the reviewer. Remember that the reviewer can only recommend changes to you whereas the final say belongs to the editor. That is why it is the editor's responsibility to revise the reviewer comments if they go against the opinion of the editor. Then this generated and partly revised email is send to you and you get a chance to produce a revised version of the manuscript.

"The reviewer comments are screened by the editor before you receive them"

You will then correct your manuscript and make a rebuttal letter with a detailed list of changes, and this is then re-submitted to the journal through the manuscript system together with a new version of your manuscript file with visible changes. Now this new submission will in most journals go directly to the editor and the editor will read it and often at this point decide immediately if the paper should be accepted or if it should go out again for a new peer review. The decision to send out for new peer review is typical if there are many changes, perhaps new statistical analyses, or new tables etc. Especially if the editor is not a specific expert in this field then the editor will need some guidance again from a new (or the same) peer reviewer. Then the paper comes back from another round of peer review and then the editor will do the same process again, copy their comments into a standard email, send it to you for new corrections and so on and you can re-submit again a new version of the paper. This can go on for maybe 2-3-4-5 different revisions but most often there will only be one revision and then the paper can be accepted. That is the typical scenario in most journals.

Now your paper is hopefully accepted for publication. You will get an email from the editor with a confirmation that the paper has now been accepted and this is of course great and you can celebrate. The next step in the editorial process is that the paper will go to a copy-editor. The copy-editor is a technical editor who will read it thoroughly for gramma errors, language, spelling, order and style of references and so on, and all these minor errors are corrected. It is not a full linguistic review, so if you are not a native English speaker and the linguistic quality of the paper is poor then you will most probably get the paper back and be asked to send it for external language revision.

After the copy-editing process at the editorial office the manuscript will go to typesetting that can be handled internally or at an external company. After typesetting you will receive the manuscript in its final form as a pdf file for proof. This is most often your only chance to correct errors. At this point you should not correct major things. Do not make new sentences or change references etc. You are only allowed to change minor errors like a wrong reference number, an error in a table, or a spelling error. So check it thoroughly at this point, especially the tables since there may be errors made by the technical editor or the graphical person.

"The copy-editor is a technical editor"

After you have approved the proof of your paper, then you send it back, typically within 24-48 hours to the editorial office again and then you are not allowed to change anything after this point. The next thing that will happen is that the paper will in most journals be published as "epub ahead of print", meaning that it will be available on the internet with a DOI-number (digital object identifier), but not with an issue number and page numbers for the specific publication, and then it will "hang" there on the Internet until there is room for it in a journal issue. Remember that the paper will already as an epub ahead of print publication be indexed in Pubmed/Medline and is therefore searchable. When it is published in a journal issue as the final publication it will of course get the full citable reference with volume, issue and page numbers.

Press releases

Many biomedical journals around the World will inform journalists about the upcoming scientific papers in the journal. They will send out press releases every week or every month depending on their frequency of publication and they will send this information to newspapers or news agencies about the upcoming papers in the journal. The press releases will not cover all articles in the journal issue, and the editor will typically choose one or two papers that are especially relevant for press releases. Then, a special summary is produced at the editorial office and it is important to say, that the summary sent as a press release is not the same as the abstract of the article. It will typically be a special summary that is produced perhaps by a journalist attached to the editorial office.

"The press release will typically be a special summary of one or two specific papers from the upcoming journal issue"

Then the special summary is sent to a journalist or a newspaper or radio or television station together with the scientific paper in question. Typically, however, the journalist at the newspaper will not necessarily read all through the scientific paper itself because it may be too much work or take too much time for him or her, but he/she will rely on the special summary sent for evaluation. That is why the editor should check the correctness of the journalistic press release summary before it is released.

The next thing that happens at the newspaper office is that if the journalist will find the paper of interest, then they will produce a news story about it. This news story will then have an embargo period because the news media are not allowed to release the story until the actual publication of the scientific paper in the journal. It is a system that is based on trust between the news media and the scientific journals and typically there are no problems about this. The newspaper will accept that they cannot release the story until the scientific paper is actually published in the scientific journal. Often the journalist on the newspaper will have the opportunity to contact the author of the scientific paper or even the editor of the journal if they want to have more information or maybe perform an interview or something like that. So the author of the paper should be prepared to be contacted by a journalist and give an interview before the paper is actually published.

"The author should be prepared to give an interview"

This is common practice in most scientific journals and the message here for you is that the newspapers will not get access to all the scientific papers in the journal, but will only receive maybe one or two stories from the journal which has been selected by the editor or the editorial team.

How do we get all data published

Undoubtedly, there is a body of research data stored in drawers around the World and these data may for various reasons never be published. This may seem harmless, but it is indeed a serious problem as it contributes to the occurrence of publication bias. In addition, it is a major ethical problem since according to the declaration of Helsinki we are obliged to publish all research data, so that patients have not participated unsuccessfully in the trials. Unfortunately, publication bias is not a rare phenomenon and you can for instance see it if you make a funnel plot in a meta-analysis, so it is indeed an important problem.

> *"Unpublished data is a serious problem"*

When all the results are not published or maybe published selectively based on the results of the trial (meaning that negative results are not published as often as they should), then clinicians do not base their treatment decisions on a proper basis. Therefore, it is very important that all gathered research data in some way are reported to the public, so that data will be available for systematic reviews and meta-analyses. The key question however is "how can we solve this problem"? We cannot force the researchers to spend time writing scientific articles if they don't have the time, the desire, or the economic opportunities to do that. On the other hand it is very important to get the data out. We therefore need some mechanisms to ensure that.

The American government has taken action here and passed the FDAAA that was updated to a final statement on September 21, 2016 (https://www.federalregister.gov/documents/2016/09/21/2016-22129/clinical-trials-registration-and-results-information-submission). This regulates the mandatory submission of summary results to www.clinicaltrials.gov if the trial involves FDA-regulated drugs or devices. It will not be the detailed results in order not to interfere with copyright for a subsequent publication in a biomedical journal, but it will give some indication of what the trial showed.

Another solution that will soon become mandatory is the obligation to share your original data with other researchers. This is recommended by the ICMJE (see e.g. http://www.nejm.org/doi/full/10.1056/NEJMe1515172) and will therefore soon find its way into author instructions in journals around the World. There are still some unsolved issues that are discussed in the editorial that was published simultaneously in all the ICMJE signature journals. This mandatory data sharing will, however, only be in place for studies that will be published (and probably only when published in certain journals to begin with) so it does not solve the problem of data lying around in drawers in offices never reaching publication. We therefore need to find other solutions to solve the problem effectively.

It may be a solution to have a publicly available repository to hold the original data from unpublished studies, but the key-question of course is who will do it and who will pay for it. Of course I don't have a solution, but a model has to be created. It could be a public archive where the investigator(s) can post a simple introduction or at least the aim of study, a short methods section and then the raw data and some kind of conclusion or at least the reason for the data not being published in a normal scientific journal. That could perhaps be a way forward and I hope that somebody will take this up. It will be an important tool against publication bias.

PUBLICATION OF RESEARCH PROTOCOLS

There are many good reasons to publish a research protocol, especially before the trial has ended. During the data analysis phase the authors will have to stick to the predefined statistical analysis plan and not for instance change primary or secondary outcomes. After publication of the research paper it will also be possible to check for this quality indicator, that the data analysis was performed as it was meant to from the design phase without post-hoc fishing expeditions. Fishing expeditions in the data analysis phase may be OK as long as they are stated that way in the paper and not included as a preplanned outcome parameter. Many ground-breaking new ideas are founded on such fishing expeditions in previous trials, but the scientific value of these findings are questionable in the paper in question since the study was not powered originally to look for these data.

> *"There are many good reasons to publish a research protocol"*

There are various options for publication of trial protocols. The best solution would probably be if clinicaltrials.gov or the other public trial databases could publish protocols in a locked/hidden version until the study is complete, and then the file could open and be readable. In essence, the protocol is put up on the web before enrolment of the first patient (so the researchers will not suddenly get good ideas depending on how the results are looking during data acquisition or analysis). This has not been implemented yet but it would be a great way to secure research integrity.

The alternative to this solution could be that all the ICMJE journals publish the research protocol together with the primary publication. However, this will not ensure that the protocol is unchanged from the original version and until it is published along with the final article. If the authors, however, have published a protocol article prior to the final trial publication, then it will replace the above-mentioned solutions if the protocol article contains a detailed plan for data analysis. Actually, the data analysis plan, the so-called statistical analysis plan, is the most important part of the protocol article. Thus, another solution would be to make the statistical analysis plan publicly available somewhere. It could be at the study registration databases or in biomedical journals as formal publications.

> *"The statistical analysis plan is the most important part of the protocol article"*

Now what types of studies should have a statistical analysis plan? So far it is only routine for the large and typically industry-sponsored studies, but it actually applies for all types of research from large interventional trials to observational studies to systematic reviews and meta-analyses. All would benefit from producing a detailed statistical analysis plan before the first data point has been collected and the statistical analysis plan should be made publicly available preferably before the final study publication.

The material for publication before the final study article could be a single pdf file of the original protocol with all the amendments, or a final protocol with its statistical analysis plan. Or alternatively in fact, it could also just be the statistical analysis plan itself without the often very large research protocol.

So you may ask, but isn't it already implemented with the mandatory trial registration? Well to some extent yes, but it is far from enough. In the current method of registration, for example at clinicaltrials.gov, you must specify various details about trial design, but the actual analysis plan is not available. Also, it is only mandatory to register clinical interventional trials, but not observational studies or systematic reviews and meta-analyses. There is a trend now to register observational studies as well as interventional trials but it is actually not mandatory. Systematic reviews and meta-analyses may be registered in the PROSPERO database, but this is also not mandatory. We therefore need a solution for all types of studies.

"The mandatory trial registration is not enough"

Right now it is impossible to say exactly how this case ends, and when there will be a solid solution, but until then we can only recommend researchers to publish protocol articles whenever possible, and to submit formal statistical analysis plans together with the original papers and have them published as supplementary material for web-only if the journals will agree to that. In the meantime, it would also be a good idea to register observational studies (on e.g. clinicaltrials.gov) and systematic reviews and meta-analyses (on PROSPERO) in a timely fashion before data acquisition.

The newest guideline from the ICMJE (Vancouver Group) has specifically recommended that for large human intervention studies the researchers should consider to publish a separate protocol article. The specific recommendation from the ICMJE is that editors receiving papers on major human intervention studies should ask to see the original study protocol or a separate statistical analysis plan for use in the review process of the journal. It is recommended that this material be made available to the public at the time of publication of the original article. This publication can be in the form of a previously published protocol article or as additional material published on the web with the final original article. Overall, it is a clear recommendation from the Vancouver group that the major human intervention studies should publish its protocol or a detailed statistical analysis plan, and this may well take the form of a previously published protocol article or made available as web-only supplementary material on the journal's website. As mentioned, I do think, however, that this recommendation should be expanded to also cover observational studies as well as systematic reviews and meta-analyses.

Why the paper was rejected

There are different reasons why a scientific paper is rejected by an editor and that is most importantly if the target audience is not correct. This means that you have submitted your paper to the wrong journal.
Of course the paper itself may not be of sufficient quality but I think that actually the most important reason for rejection, at least for immediate rejection, is when the target audience is incorrect. You have to think about this carefully when you choose your journal, so for instance if you are writing a paper about a molecule receptor or something like that, then it will usually not fit the target audience for one of the big general medical journals like the Lancet or JAMA.

> *"The most important reason for immediate rejection is when the target audience is incorrect"*

Then the editor will also look at the readability of your paper. If it is very difficult to read then it will be returned to you (or immediately rejected), because it has to be easy to read and easy to understand. The article has to be written in very clear language and it has to be easy to follow the text. The general trend in scientific publication is that the language has to be easy to read. A positive by-product is that it will actually also be easier for you to write the paper using easy language instead of using numerous difficult words and complicated sentence structures. The reason for the editor's preference of easy language is that there are many sources of information out there available for the scientific reader, so they have to stay onboard and read your paper. If your language is too complicated, then they will simply skip the paper and find something else to read. Thus, the scientific article has to be easy to read with clear and few messages using easy language - not fancy scientific language - and then you will probably have an easier task of getting your paper accepted for publication.

> *"The article has to be written in clear language and it has to be easy to follow the text"*

The paper has to have a clear message, meaning a clear hypothesis with a clear aim of study, and thereby a clear message to the reader. It is not common nowadays to see papers with many different hypotheses and different aims and sub-aims making the paper extremely difficult to read and in fact also very difficult for you to write. So, keep it reasonably simple and preferably have only one or very few hypotheses and aims of study. If your original study design included several hypotheses, then you should consider to split the study in two or more separate publications each with a specific study aim. This will make it much easier to read and is therefore positive for the reader. This phenomenon is sometimes called "salami-slicing", which has a negative sound to it, but as you see it is actually a positive thing from the reader's point of view. And that is what is important here! We have to please the reader in order to get our papers read.

> *"The paper has to have a clear message"*

If you ignore "instructions to authors" that is also a typical reason why your paper will be rejected by the editorial office. If instructions say that you have to use a certain style for references or that the length of the manuscript should be within a certain limit, then you of course have to comply. These instructions are not made only for other authors than you. They are general rules that have to be followed by all authors.

Another thing that the editor will consider is the originality of the paper. Is this something new? Is it a good story for the readers? The paper has to attract readers to the journal so that revenue will increase and hopefully also the journal impact factor when the article gets cited by other researchers. Preferably the paper should represent an important step forward and be a first time publication.

Another thing that is considered by the editor is the reproducibility of the study meaning "is it so easy to follow your experiment that it can actually be reproduced by other researchers?" – this is also important.

A critical situation is when you are replying to editor and peer reviewers in a rebuttal letter. I remember a case we had where I as an editor wrote to the authors that they had to shorten the paper 10% and delete a figure. Then the authors responded that they would not do that. Now what do you think happened? Of course the paper was rejected. So, it is very important to comply with the changes requested by the editor and also to comply in detail with the instructions to authors.

In the revision phase you should as far as possible comply with the requests for changes made by the peer reviewers. As discussed above in the chapter about handling revisions you are of course allowed to argue against suggested changes if the reviewer has obviously misunderstood something, but as a general rule it is a good idea to take on the mindset of complying with as much as possible. This will increase your chance of getting your paper accepted for publication.

> *"It is a good idea to comply with the requests for changes made by the editor and the reviewers"*

To round up I would say that the most important factor for your paper being rejected is that you have chosen the wrong journal. So look at the journal's aim, look at the target audience, and from that you can decide on the most appropriate journal for your scientific article. Comply with instructions to authors and to comments from peer reviewers and the editor in the revision phase. Finally, focus on readability so that everybody can follow the text without slowing the speed of reading and without making the reader frustrated.

COMMITTEE ON PUBLICATION ETHICS

All researchers should know about this committee and their freely available material.

As a new researcher (or even as an old researcher) you may not even know that this committee exists. It is a committee that was established back in 1997 by a group of journal editors and now has more than 10,000 members worldwide, both journal editors and also other individuals with an interest in publication ethics. The reason why I think that you should know about the existence of this committee is that they have freely available fantastic flow-charts where you can find answers to different questions on publication ethics, authorship issues etc. This means that if you experience one of these problems in your research career and if your paper is under consideration by a journal, then you should know that the journal editor will go to this exact resource and look up how to handle it. So why not be prepared for that and look it up yourself before it goes to an authorship dispute or a case of fraud suspicion with possible article retraction etc.

"www.publicationethics.org"

You can find all the available information on www.publicationethics.org where everything is free of charge. It is a great resource. This committee are developing flow-charts covering different scenarios. Currently, they have these flowcharts available:

How to respond to whistle blowers
- Responding to Whistle blowers - Concerns Raised Directly
- Responding to Whistle blowers - Concerns Raised via Social Media

Changes in Authorship
- Corresponding author requests addition of extra author before publication
- Corresponding author requests removal of author before publication
- Request for addition of extra author after publication
- Request for removal of author after publication
- Suspected guest, ghost or gift authorship
- How to spot authorship problems

Conflict of Interest
- What to do if a reviewer suspects undisclosed conflict of interest in a submitted manuscript
- What to do if a reader suspects undisclosed conflict of interest in a published article

What to do if you suspect an ethical problem
- What to do if you suspect an ethical problem with a submitted manuscript

What to do if you suspect fabricated data
- Suspected fabricated data in a submitted manuscript
- Suspected fabricated data in a published manuscript

What to do if you suspect a reviewer has appropriated an author's idea or data
- What to do if you suspect a reviewer has appropriated an author's idea or data

What to do if you suspect plagiarism
- Suspected plagiarism in a submitted manuscript
- Suspected plagiarism in a published manuscript

What to do if you suspect redundant (duplicate) publication
- Suspected redundant publication in a submitted manuscript
- Suspected redundant publication in a published manuscript

In these flowcharts you will see that COPE (that is The Committee on Publication Ethics referred to as COPE in daily speaking) will guide the journal editors on how to handle these problems. Very often it will require some sensitive correspondence, first with the authors and if this does not solve the problem then the correspondence will go to the chiefs of these authors meaning head of department or faculty dean or something like that. Always the journal editor will ask politely about the potential problem and depending on the answer then the process will continue. For instance, if there is a request for addition of an author after the paper has been submitted, that will require a signature from all the other authors on the paper on the byline and of course also a statement from this new author that he or she has fulfilled the four authorship criteria from the ICMJE. So, you can see that if you are about to encounter a problem about your publication you can go to this resource on www.publicationethics.org and find an answer or a solution to the problem hopefully before it gets out of hand. That is why knowing about COPE is a good advice for you. I can assure you that many if not all journal editors know about this resource and they use them. So, go there, study it, and hopefully this will produce better research ethics in the future.

Part 4: Peer review

TYPES OF PEER REVIEW

It is important to know the roles of the different people involved in the process. First of all, the journal is owned by a publisher, so the publisher will hire and fire the editor and will decide the overall aim of the journal. The editor is the head of daily operations of the journal and is usually the highest ranked person in the editorial office. The editor has the final decision about acceptance or rejection of a submitted paper.

This means that the peer reviewer can give suggestions to the editor. As a peer reviewer you can give advice that the paper should be accepted or rejected or revised and resubmitted, but you have actually nothing to say whatsoever about acceptance or rejection. This also means that in your peer-review comments to authors you should not say anything about acceptance or rejection. You can only say that directly to the editor in the special section of the peer review comments where you write confidential comments to the editor.

> *"The editor has the final decision about acceptance or rejection of a submitted paper"*

There are different types of peer review. You can have a double blind peer review, a single blind, or an open peer review. In the double blind system the reviewer does not know the identity of the author and the author does not know the identity of the reviewer. Some journals will use single-blind peer review meaning that the peer reviewer will know the identity of the author, but the author will not know the identity of the reviewer. Then, finally there is the open system, where everybody's name is open, so the author will know who performed the peer review and of course the peer reviewer will also know the author names.

> *"Peer review can be double blind, single blind, or open"*

Typically in smaller journals or smaller communities it is normal to use double blind peer review because the scientific community may be so small that everybody more or less know each other. Thus, in these smaller communities an open system for peer review may cause problems if for instance a younger peer reviewer will give tough criticism to a paper written by one of the professors in the area. So in order to prevent bias in the peer review process it may be advisable to use blinded review in smaller research communities.

The most often used system for international journals is probably the single-blind system where only the identity of the peer reviewer is kept secret to the author. Open peer review is typically used in journals and communities that are global, meaning that it will be easier to find a peer reviewer that does not have any conflicts of interest against the author and vice versa. Sometimes these journals, like for instance the BMJ, will publish (electronically) all the details of the peer review process, all the comments, rebuttal letters etc. This is not common, however, and usually all the correspondence in the peer review process is kept confidential (see chapter below about confidentiality).

> *"The most often used system for international journals is probably the single-blind system"*

Then there is a newer system called post-publication peer review and this is really groundbreaking. It means, that the paper is checked by the editorial office and by the editor before it is taken in and then the paper is without formal peer review put out in the open on the Internet and actually as a publication that will be indexed in databases like PubMed etc. After publication it is open for peer review, so peer review comments will come in after publication and then the authors may change the paper afterwards and then publish a second version, and then a third version and so on. An example of a journal, which is running like that, is the F1000Research. This system is really interesting and if the research communities accept it we may see even newer ways for publication of research findings. Who knows, maybe future peer review will be something on social media. The possibilities are certainly not fully explored yet. There are pros and cons, but one advantage is that it will ensure that everything is published immediately so there is no lack time for publication. This is very interesting. We will have to see where this will end eventually.

How to perform peer review

The journal will typically send you an email asking you to do a peer review and then you will have to decide if you can do it. You may first become a little worried and maybe doubt if you are good enough for this honorable task. To this I will say that of course you are good enough. Very often peer review is also a way of giving critical feedback from an unbiased reader, meaning a reader that do not have to be an expert in the field, but will give valuable comments to the author (and editor) about the general readability of the paper. The next thing you may worry is whether you need to prepare or study and the answer to this is definitely no. You need to know about research methodology and then have common sense. Of course it will be nice if you know details within the field of research but you do not need to be an expert. To make your decision to accept the task the only material that you have is typically the email from the Journal including perhaps the abstract of the paper and then you have to decide.

"You do not need to be an expert"

The thing you should decide upon now is first of all whether you have the time needed to do it. That is the most important thing. Then secondly you will also need to decide if you have any potential conflicts of interest against this paper or the authors. If you have conflicts of interest you should of course decline to review the paper. You are not allowed to do it if you have any potential conflicts of interest, and only accept if you have the time to do it within the next week.

Now you will start the process. You get access to the full paper from the journal after pressing an acceptance link in the email. In my opinion the best way to do it is to start with a very fast reading (maximum 10 minutes) of the whole article from beginning to end without making any comments or any notes. When you do this you should consider yourself to be the general reader of the journal and decide if you understand what it is about. After this initial reading I usually read it again, and then during this second reading I make notes on paper. Remember the first reading is only very fast reading just to get an overview of what it is all about, and then the second time it takes a little bit more time and then you write comments and notes on the papers on the way.

> *"Start with a very fast reading and make notes during the second reading"*

Then you have to sit back a little and think about this article. The first thing you have to consider is if the journal in question is the right place for publication – if the target audience is correct. This is perhaps the most important thing to consider because if for instance the paper is about a detailed veterinary research question and it is submitted to a clinical medical journal, then it may not be the best place to publish it. So you should consider this very carefully. The second thing you have to think about is the originality of the study, meaning if it is the first time it has been shown or if it duplication of previous work. Duplication work is of value and can certainly be published, but it will somehow of course lower the quality and maybe the impact of the study. So, think about this and inform the editor in the section for confidential comments to editor. Then, the third thing you have to think about is the readability of the paper. If the language is too complicated and if it is a difficult design with different hypotheses and aims and sub-aims, then it may not be a good idea to publish that article. Think about the easiness of understanding of the paper. Think about the reader.

"Consider issues like target audience, originality and readability"

Now you come to the actual writing of your review comments. This is of course done online in the manuscript management system or whatever it is called. There are dedicated text fields to fill out including comments to the author and confidential comments to the editor. In these confidential comments to the editor you write your thoughts about your general assessment of the paper. Is the target audience correct, are there potential problems with conflict of interests or bias or are there any issues of other ongoing research in the field. You should also give some thoughts about the clinical importance of the study, because the editor may not be fully updated here. An editor cannot of course know everything about all clinical areas so you can write here your thoughts about the clinical importance. Then you will give some general comments about language and grammar, spelling, and the use of references. Finally, in this field you can give your recommendations to the editor about acceptance, revision, or rejection. You do not have the final decision here, but you can give your recommendations to the editor. That is something that the editor would most often like to see.

"You give confidential comments to the editor and general and detailed comments to the author"

Now, in another text field you give the comments to authors. It is normal routine to first give a very short summary of the paper in the first paragraph, maybe 2 or 3 lines. Be positive, be friendly and be constructive in your criticism, and you should not reveal your identity. After your general comments in the first paragraph you will give detailed comments to authors and in this process you now will use your notes from the second reading of the paper. It is a very good idea to use a numbered list because when the author makes his or her rebuttal letter then he or she can use the same numbers. In this field, where you give comments directly to the authors, you should not say anything about recommending acceptance, revision or rejection.

Now you are done, it is not difficult and it is fun and you will also learn a lot yourself while doing peer review. So I can fully recommend that you accept the task if you have the time to do it.

Peer review good behavior

If you are peer reviewing a scientific paper you are not allowed to discuss it with anyone outside the editorial process except if the editor expressly authorizes it. The material is considered confidential information and similarly the peer reviewer is not allowed to store copies of the reviewed manuscript or to apply knowledge from such papers outside of the editorial process.

In your peer review you should of course give an objective assessment of the available facts and thereby completely disregard your personal or professional bias. Therefore, if you do have a conflict of interest for instance in the specific research field or especially against the specific authors or the author group, then it is important to refuse to review the paper. You simply tell the editor about the situation and there is no problem about that. Then you can skip this peer review and the editor will choose another one. Very few journals use the ICMJE conflict of interest form for peer reviewers, but the authors have to fill that out. The ICMJE form could obviously also be used for peer reviewers as well as editors but it is often not the case. If the journal does not require you to complete the ICMJE form as a peer reviewer you could then just yourself inform the editor if you have any relevant potential conflicts of interest.

The feedback from the peer reviewer should be constructive and not too negative, but of course you have to give constructive feedback and this can sometimes be slightly negative. You can help by keeping a good tone and not use unnecessary hard language in your feedback for the authors. There is absolutely no reason to be rude. You could point out all the positive aspects of the work first and then in your point to point criticism you can go through different aspects, which of course may be considered to be negative, but if you use a constructive tone it will not be a problem. You can then give the authors the opportunity to improve the manuscript in the following revision rounds.

> *"Do not use unnecessary hard language in your feedback."*

If you suspect plagiarism or maybe even data fabrication, which is extremely rare, then you should tell that to the editor of course. It is often the peer reviewer who gets the suspicion because he or she is typically better informed in the subject field compared with the editor. In these cases you should tell the editor about your suspicion in the feedback form (confidential comments to editor). For peer review there are two distinctive fields, one only for the editor and one for the author, so this is information that should go only to the editor.

Depending on the peer review system that is employed by the journal you should also be very careful not to expose yourself in the peer review comments. If the journal uses single blind or double blind peer review then the author is not allowed to know your identity. Thus, you should be careful not to expose yourself, meaning that you should not actually write who you are and your judgment should not reflect your specific field of expertise if for instance you are the only one in the world who could know some specific information and if you put that down in your review, then it is obvious for the author who you actually are.

"If peer review is blinded you should not expose yourself"

It is not OK to ask the authors to cite specific articles in their reference list and especially when it is your own paper that you ask them to cite. So, please do not say anything about specific references that you want to be included in the reference list. This implies also that you should not ask the authors to have a positive attitude towards your work and a negative attitude towards competitors.

When you have performed your peer review and sent your comments to the editorial office, then the editor will read your assessment. A good editor will of course read the comments for authors very carefully and also revise it, because sometimes a reviewer may suggest that the author should delete a figure or include new material, and if the editor actually does not want that then he or she has to take care of that, meaning revise/change the reviewer comments, before sending the comments to the authors. Unfortunately, this does not always happen, and sometimes it creates confusion for the author about what he or she should do.

Confidentiality in the Review Process

A basic rule in all journal offices around the World is to use full confidentiality regarding the submitted scientific articles. This means that persons involved in the editorial process cannot speak to others about an ongoing evaluation of a scientific paper. There is a full secrecy agreement among all the involved persons – from secretaries to peer reviewers and editors. It is the same level of secrecy agreement that we use every day in our clinical work with patients. Journal editors keep this principle of confidentiality very high.

Similarly, it is important that authors adhere to this professional secrecy agreement and thus do not tell anyone about their results before the article is published. Of course you can present the results at a scientific congress as a lecture, and have an abstract published in the congress book or present a poster, but a detailed report of the results to a third party is not OK. The risk is that a journal will regard this as a prior publication and it therefore means that you will not be able to get your paper accepted for publication.

Also the external evaluators in the peer review process are subject to strict confidentiality. They must not use information from the articles in their own research, or talk about the results to other people. This principle of confidentiality for assessors applies whether using open or blinded peer review.

"All involved persons have strict confidentiality regarding the scientific paper"

However, there are no formal sanctions if confidentiality is broken, but it will probably mean that it will be difficult in the future to get approval of the reviewer's own articles, and of course this person will not be used as a reviewer in the future.

There are exceptions to this general rule of confidentiality. The four exceptions are:

1) If the journal wishes to prepare an invited commentary or an editorial for simultaneous publication with the original article. Then the manuscript of the original paper is shared with the author of the editorial or commentary.
2) If the results have great widespread clinical importance, meaning that it can potentially save human lives as soon as it gets public, and in this case, the journal may choose to publish the results or the conclusion before the final article can be published.
3) Results can be published in a summary format on clinicaltrials.gov before the paper gets out. This is accepted by most journals because the Vancouver group has supported it in their recommendations.
4) You can present your results at a congress or scientific meeting as a lecture or poster. Just be careful not to

provide handouts with detailed results since a journal editor could interpret this as a prior publication.

Thus, you can as an author assume that your article will be kept secret to all but those who are directly involved in the editorial process. This applies until the paper is published either on the net or in print. And you should do the same.

Part 5: Closing

When you have finished your scientific paper it is fascinating to follow its way through the editorial process. The purpose of the present book was therefore to give you some insight into this work flow because it may actually help you in the writing process because you can take certain issues into account before you submit your paper to a scientific journal.

First of all it is very important to follow the ICMJE criteria for authorship and also to know about other critical issues on authorship. You have therefore learned in this book that the order of authors in the byline have some unwritten rules attached to it, that it is not so important how many authors are placed in the byline as long as they all fulfill the ICMJE criteria for authorship, and that the use of group authorship is probably on the return. It is self-explanatory that a paper should only have one corresponding author and I strongly suggest that you create an ORCID ID so that your name will not be confused with the name of other authors. Finally, author disputes should preferably be prevented and taken care of before they even occur, but if they do occur there are some help to obtain but importantly this help will not come from the editorial office because author disputes have to be settled by the author group before submission of the article.

When you submit your paper you should give attention to the cover letter, which is a personal letter from you to the editor. This is important because you here get the chance to explain to the editor why your paper is a fantastic piece of work, and why the editor should accept it for publication. If you get the paper back from the editorial office with suggestions for changes made by the editor and peer reviewers and you thereby get a chance to revise it and re-submit, then you should handle this using a firm template for the rebuttal letter. The editor gets many of these rebuttal letters so it will make the editor's work easier if you use the same template every time.

I hope that I have explained the editorial process for you and especially explained why a paper is typically rejected because you undoubtedly will experience this every once in a while. The main reason for rejection is probably that the target audience is wrong, so you should consider this issue carefully before submitting your paper to a journal. Other important reasons are of course the scientific quality of your article as well as the linguistic quality level.

If you experience a problem that resembles editorial problems then it is actually a good idea, even though you are not an editor yourself, to consult the flow charts at the COPE website (www.publicationethics.org).

Finally, you will certainly be asked to be a peer reviewer at some point and I have therefore discussed the process of peer review in this book as well. I hope that this will be helpful for you.

Other books in this series

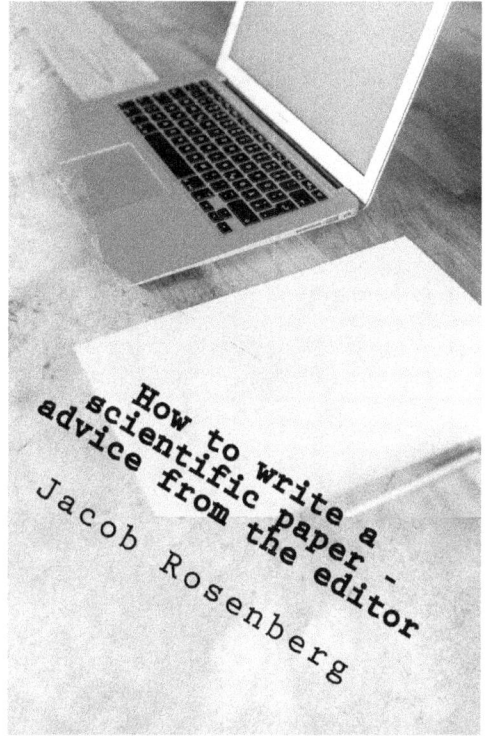

How to write a scientific paper: advice from the editor
Ultimate Researcher's Guide Series, Volume 1.

Available as paperback and kindle edition on all Amazon platforms.

Notes

contact

www.biomedicalpublishing.com

www.ingramcontent.com/pod-product-compliance
Lightning Source LLC
Chambersburg PA
CBHW061149180526
45170CB00002B/689